MW01100474

Driving Your Woman
Wild in Bed

Yes

Driving
Your Woman
Wild in Bed

Yes

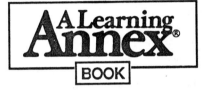

COMPILED AND EDITED BY

Susan Wright

A Citadel Press Book
Published by Carol Publishing Group

Carol Publishing Group Edition, 1995

Copyright © 1992 by Susan Wright
All rights reserved. No part of this book may be reproduced in any form,
except by a newspaper or magazine reviewer who wishes to quote brief
passages in connection with a review.

A Citadel Press Book
Published by Carol Publishing Group
Citadel Press is a registered trademark of Carol Communications, Inc.

Editorial Offices: 600 Madison Avenue, New York, NY 10022
Sales & Distribution Offices: 120 Enterprise Avenue, Secaucus, NJ 07094
In Canada: Canadian Manda Group, One Atlantic Avenue, Suite 105
Toronto, Ontario, M6K 3E7

Queries regarding rights and permissions should be addressed to:
Carol Publishing Group, 600 Madison Avenue, New York, NY 10022

Manufactured in the United States of America
10 9 8 7 6 5 4

Carol Publishing Group books are available at special discounts
for bulk purchases, sales promotions, fund raising, or
educational purposes. Special editions can also be created to
specifications. For details contact: Special Sales Department,
Carol Publishing Group, 120 Enterprise Ave., Secaucus, NJ 07094

Library of Congress Cataloging-in-Publication Data

Driving your woman wild in bed / A Learning Annex book
    Compiled and edited by Susan Wright.
    Previously published as The Learning Annex Guide to Driving
    Your Woman Wild in Bed.
    p. cm.
"A Citadel Press book."
ISBN 0-8065-1331-4
1. Sex instruction for men. 2. Women–Sexual behavior.
I. Wright, Susan (Susan G.) II. Learning Annex (Firm)
III. Title: Guide to driving your woman wild in bed.
HQ36.L43   1992
613.9'6'024041—dc20   92-9663
                                                  CIP

Contents

Driving Your Woman
Wild in Bed

1 | *Are You Good in Bed ?*

I'm sure you want to be good in bed. But how do you know whether you are good or not?

Well, here are some answers: *How to Drive Your Woman Wild in Bed*. And though this book is written for men *about* women, your ultimate success depends on the response of your lover. Try sharing this book with your lover; talking about sex is an excellent way to discover her true feelings and desires.

Of course, no book can cover everything about the sexual experience, but these tips will give you and your lover a good start on a relationship filled with wonderful sex.

First Things First

The two most important things to remember about your lover are:

1. For a woman, sex is an emotional as well a physical experience.
2. To keep the spark alive, sex should be a variety of experiences and never a routine.

If you understand these two points and incorporate them into your sexual encounters, you'll have a good chance of driving your woman wild in bed.

Go EASy on the first part of point 1 or else you run the risk of being Rock SiMPLy in the AMAtuor video

Emotional and Physical

It isn't what you know about sex or what you can do as far as any technique is concerned that will drive your lover

3

wild in bed. For most women, sex is an emotional *and* physical experience, and a great lover will accept and nurture both of these aspects.

Men tend to focus more on the physical side of sex—technique, skill, physical beauty—and often neglect the emotional side of the experience. This lack of balance is the difference between a man who can drive his woman wild in bed and one who can't.

Instead of thinking about your performance, concentrate on your feelings. What is it you like about your lover? What does she seem to like about you? If there is no affection between you, then you probably shouldn't be having a sexual encounter with this woman.

When you involve your feelings, then your emotional relationship with your lover will lead you to do what comes naturally. You'll react in erotic, physical ways not because you feel you ought to, but because you want to. That is how you satisfy your lover in bed.

Never a Routine

You will be a great lover only if you are enthusiastic about widening the scope of your erotic experience. If you genuinely wish to come together with your lover and create a mutually enjoyable experience, it won't matter if you aren't entirely clear about all physical details of sex.

Experiment and be open about sex with your lover. There is no one method, no perfect position, no sequence of moves that will enable you to be great in bed. This is not a 1–2–3 process. Your sexual encounters should be an exciting and varied experience. But, don't make the mistake of mechanically performing lots of little "sexy" things without thinking of how and when you should do them.

2 | *Romance*

What does a woman really want in a sexual relationship? She wants romance.

"Romance" simply means that a woman wants to be more than just a sexual partner to you. She wants to be caressed and kissed with affection. She wants to talk to you.

When your lover thinks of sex with you, she'll often focus on being close to you, feeling your warmth pressing against her skin, breaking boundaries and invading each other's space, becoming one with you in an act of physical union. *she thinks of that ol BiG fAt HAIRY MONSTER!*

Your lover also wants *verbal* as well as physical confirmation that she is important to you, that you respect and admire her, and that you want to please her. It's important that you *tell* your lover these things—simply *thinking* them will do nothing to improve your sexual relationship. *TALK is good*

As is true for many men, it may simply be a lack of a good role model that inhibits your romantic behavior. But don't you want your lover to listen to you, be there for you, and share her life with you?

THIS book is NEArly not as dim as I hoped

Touching

If you only touch your lover when you want sex, you ll never create a comfortable, contact-filled relationship.

In addition, if you always respond to your lover's touch by wanting to take it to sexual intercourse, your lover will stop touching you. You absolutely must give your lover hugs and caresses outside of sex. *Yes that's Right Not*

When she gives you a good-bye kiss, don't just make it a ritual peck. Stroke her hair, hold her hand, or cuddle with her on the couch while you watch TV. Caress her breast as she passes by you, rub her buttocks, give her a long, sweet kiss. Then let her go her own way. Remember, don't push it to sex every time. *Yes that sounds good too*

Attention

Do little things for your lover, both in and out of bed. Even silly, romantic things—gifts, notes, flowers—will truly please your lover and go a long way toward reaffirming that she is important to you. Surprise her by bringing home ice cream or tickets to a play or a movie you can watch together. But don't stop there. You can also leave her sex- or love-notes, play strip poker, make bets with sexual payoffs, buy her erotic gifts and clothes, or take sexy Polariod pictures of her. These little things show that you think about her and care enough about her to consider just how you can surprise, please, and satisfy her. *BFHC*

Don't forget to show her attention in front of other people, as well. When you introduce her to your friends, show by your smile and attention that you're fond of your lover. Affirming your bond in public will earn you a place in her heart.

Talking

You have probably fantasized hundreds of different ways to begin a sexual encounter. So have women. The biggest difference between men's and women's fantasies is that for women, the ideal foreplay starts with conversation.

This doesn't mean you have to be a silver-tongued Don Juan. It does mean that if you are attracted to a woman, and she has reciprocated that attraction, your words can often do more to give her pleasure than any sort of touching or smoldering glances you manage to accomplish.

Talking doesn't mean discussing the day-to-day details of your life. Talk to her about your future, your dreams (past and present), your ideas of what makes a good relationship. Ask your lover about her dreams and plans. She'll be stunned by your sensitivity.

THAT WOULD MAKE me SICK

3 | *Talking About Sex*

The idea of mysterious sex—with a strange, willing woman unexpectedly making advances to you—is very compelling for most men. If you are faced with such a situation, and feel comfortable and eager to go along with it, by all means have fun. But this sort of wordless approach is wrong for most of your sexual encounters, particularly if you want to have sex with a woman more than once.

Most people, especially men, are too shy to start talking about sex. Many men even think it's not important to talk about sex, and they never try to overcome their inhibitions. But if you want to drive your lover wild in bed, you must discuss sex with her. *Yes more talk Diety talk*

Generally, in terms of sexual excitement, men are more visually attuned, while women are much more verbally responsive. If you ignore your responsibility to enter into sexual conversations with your lover, how will you ever know if you are fulfilling her needs?

Even a man who is very comfortable with his lover somtimes has trouble discussing his needs and desires, as well as those of his lover. Probably the best time to be open to sexual conversation is while you are actually having intercourse. Ask her, "Does this feel good?" Tell her when she's making you feel good. If it's something you don't like, just caution her, "That hurts," or more specific instructions like sighing out, "Lower, yes...." or pleading, "More, darling!"

After sex, when you are both holding each other and

satisfied, is the perfect time to talk about sex. Tell her what felt great, what you would like to do to her, how much you care about her.

Though it might seem to be the most natural option, you don't have to be physically intimate when you talk about sex. Some people find it easier if they are both dressed and in a cool, calm frame of mind.

You can use a number of indirect methods of opening a discussion—such as books, movies, games, etc. But you won't get anywhere until you actually *say* what you feel. Hints and innuendo just don't work well when it comes to sex. And don't tease her about sexual things she does or doesn't do. Teasing is *not* talking. She will think you're laughing at her and will simply be more inhibited.

Asking your lover questions is a good way to open the conversation. "What do you like about making love to me?" "What would you like to try?" "What would you like more of?" "Less of?"

If you dive on in and start talking, you'll find that it gets easier as you go along. Both of you need to keep an open mind, and not get sidetracked into other areas of your relationship while talking about sex.

Criticism

It's not a good idea to start off criticizing something that your lover does while you're having sex. Tell her what feels good first. Tell here what is sexy about her. Then, she won't feel attacked if you mention some things that make you uncomfortable.

If your lover has a criticism of you, don't assume she thinks you're not a good lover. If you listen and learn from her suggestions, you will be a better lover for this partner as well as any future partners.

Make sure you don't fall into the trap of talking about sex only when you have a problem. Discussion should be used to enhance your sexual experience with your lover. If your discussions are always negative, then eventually neither one of you will want to talk about sex, much less have it.

Jealousy

Your lover may want to talk more about past relationships more than you do. It is a personal decision if you decide to participate in a discussion about past lovers. It is best in the long run not to delve into the sexual particulars about past lovers. Whatever you do, don't compare her to a past lover, even if the comparison is a good one. She'll wonder, and ask, what she's *bad* at compared with that lover. No woman appreciates being judged and she knows that if you do it to one lover, you'll do it to another.

When it comes to being jealous of your lover, she may be flattered at first. But, if your jealousy is prolonged or intense, she will eventually come to the conclusion that you are insecure. You'll only end up irritating her. The way to win your lover's respect is by respecting and trusting her.

If you both agree to have a monogamous, exclusive relationship, you each have the responsibility of making it clear that your partner is the most important person of the opposite sex in your life. You should make it a point to tell her what you like about her—throughout the relationship, not just in the beginning.

Inhibitions

Ideally, sex should be a welcome and fulfilling part of life. When people consider sex a natural thing, they are able to communicate it more easily and are able to enjoy a broader range of experience in their sexual encounters.

If you or your lover have inhibitions about certain sex acts, or are uncomfortable with sexuality, then in order to have a fulfilling sexual experience you must talk to one another. This will be contrary to your natural inclinations, but you must make your feelings known to keep from hurting your lover's sensibilities. Talking about sex is the only way to increase the satisfaction of both partners.

You and your lover needn't engage in acts that are incompatible with your values, but you owe it to each other to explain the way you feel. You also owe it to each other to not judge each other's preferences as immoral or perverted. Just as you could not completely understand sexual intercourse when you were a virgin, you won't be able to understand, and therefore judge, any variation you haven't tried. If you can keep an open mind, and are able to trust your partner, there's a good chance you'll be surprised by your own reaction.

4 | *Giving and Receiving*

Sex should be a combination of both giving and receiving.

A man who always wants to "receive" will never be a good lover. If you only think about your own pleasure, it's likely you'll be interfering with your lover's. You have to stop worrying about yourself and your own pleasure, and start thinking about what you can do to give your lover pleasure. You have to think of what you can do to make her feel wanted and loved and good in order to drive her wild in bed. YES WILD

On the other hand, if you *only* think about your lover and her pleasure, then you could end up ignoring your own wants and needs.

There are several different reasons why you may want to always "give"—perhaps it gives you a sense of control, or you may feel so inhibited about being intimate with a woman that you detach your feelings from the lovemaking process. Or, you may have the mistaken notion that the way to drive your woman wild in bed is by catering to her every desire. This is not a bad idea...but by focusing entirely on your lover, you're depriving her of an essential part of the sexual experience—giving to you. Some women may even become inhibited, feeling as if they're being watched and every orgasm counted. No woman likes to be used by a man's ego, as he proves to himself that he is a good lover.

A good sexual relationship includes both giving and receiving—and it can actually be a good way to vary your sexual encounters. Don't keep a mental tally sheet of who's

expect

done what to whom. Don't expert fellatio every time you give her cunnilingus. And don't feel as if you have to even up the score when she gives you a massage. Sex is a mutual act, and the giving and receiving should be joined together in a continuous, harmonious flow.

Learn from Your Lover

No one can learn how to be good in bed without help. Men and women need to learn together. And while it seems natural for a man to introduce a woman to new sexual experiences, most men make the mistake of believing that once they have lost their virginity, they should be more technically proficient and knowledgeable than the women they have sex with. This attitude will keep you from being good in bed.

The only way you can drive your woman wild in bed is by incorporating her experience into your sexual relationship. If your lover has had more experience, then you should consider yourself very lucky. This is a chance to expand your sexual horizons, and only by a welcome acceptance of her knowledge will you be able to drive her wild in bed. And even if your lover is less experienced than you, she will have her own contributions to make—just as you give something special to a more experienced partner.

Your primary responsibility in a sexual encounter is to be open. It is a mutual experience, and it will only be complete if there is an exchange made between both lovers.

Teaching Your Lover

If your lover is hesitant about doing something sexual, it probably isn't that she has an aversion to it. It's more likely that she's simply never done it before, and she doesn't want to be awkward or bad at it. *I'll be gentle with you*

You have a wonderful opportunity when this occurs. You

can broaden your lover's sexual experience. First, you should be very open with your lover—explain what it is that you would like to do, how you would do it, and what it feels like. Mystery and sex are a compelling couple, but when you are introducing your lover to something she is unsure of, you owe it to both of you to be as explicit as possible.

You should never pressure your lover. Give her time to adjust to the new idea. After all, you want her to want this. If she trusts you enough to be intimate with you, she will continue to trust you as long as it's clear that you don't expect anything from her.

5 | *The Female Body*

Only by knowing a woman's body can you please it.

Be admiring and friendly toward your lover's body, including her sex organs. Too many men simply ignore their lover's genitals, except during penetration. It might help to know that a woman's sex organs aren't that different from yours. The clitoris and the penis are composed of the same type of sensitive tissue. Your scrotum and her outer lips (labia majora) are also similar. Your lover's genitals aren't foreign territory, but something you already know a lot about.

The Vulva

The world *vulva* simply means those parts of the woman's sex organs that can be seen. The mons veneris (mount of Venus), the outer lips (labia majora) and inner lips (labia minora), the vaginal opening, the urethra, and the clitoris.

The mons veneris is the padding of flesh over the public bone. It is covered by strands of public hair. The mons is remarkably responsible to stroking and pressure.

The outer lips protect everything else. In some woman, these folds of flesh are thick and meet over her sex organ. In others, the lips simply lie to either side of the sex organs. Each woman is different, just as each man's penis is slightly different.

The inner lips are very tender and delicate. During arousal, they are usually moistened by vaginal lubricant.

15

The urethra is positioned within the inner lips, just below the clitoris and above the entrance to the vagina. Don't ever insert anything into the urethra. This area is sensitive, and is an entirely personal thing whether it is pleasurable to your lover for the urethra to be touched. For some women, it is actually painful when it is handled.

The Clitoris

The small hood that forms the joining of the outer lips protects the clitoris. This is the magic spot, the place you want to know about. Any man who understands and respects the clitoris will be considered a good lover.

Like an iceberg, only the tip of the clitoris can be seen. Under the hood, it looks like a tiny pink pea. When a woman is aroused, the clitoris fills with blood just like a man's penis, pushing slightly out of the protective hood.

It is the stimulation of the clitoris that leads to female climax. The action of a man's penis entering the vagina pulls on the inner lips, stimulating the clitoris by pulling on its hood. The man's pubic bone rubbing against the clitoris also creates arousal. But don't think you have to grind into a woman to make her climax. If you stimulate her clitoris before intercourse, the natural contact will be sufficient. No !

So how do you find the clitoris without a road map? Especially when some women themselves are unaware of exactly where their clitoris is and what it does?

The clitoris is at the top of the sexual organs. It is the first thing you come to, directly in the center, between the outer lips. It feels like a soft ridge of flesh with a dent in it, positioned just above the inner lips.

The easiest way to stimulate the clitoris is to simply rub the ridge side to side. You can feel it slip back and forth beneath your fingers. Or you can put your finger in the dent, then gently rub or tug the small hood of flesh toward her belly button. She'll love you forever.

Many women will assist you when you get close to the clitoris. Even a clumsy attempt will arouse them, and they will want you to hit the right spot. Pay attention to any movements your lover makes, because it's almost an instinctual act for her to try to draw your hand to the clitoris.

The Vagina

It's a mistake to think of the vagina as a hole. The vagina is a hollow ring of muscles, approximately four inches long. (And all this time you've been worried that your six-inch penis isn't enough to satisfy your lover! It's more than enough.)

The upper and lower ends of the vagina are the narrowest. The opening of the vagina is partially covered by the labia minora, the inner lips which become engorged with blood during intercourse. In most virgins (women who have not had sexual intercourse) the actual opening of the vagina is partially closed by a thin fold of tissue known as the hymen. Nowadays, the hymen is often broken when a girl first begins to use tampons.

The cervix of the uterus connects to the front of the inner end of the vagina. The cervix is a firm, mushroom-shaped bump. The small dent in the center is an opening that leads to the uterus, where a woman is impregnated.

There are no glands inside the vagina. The mucus that lubricates the vaginal cavity mostly comes from the uterus through the cervix. However, the cells in the lining produce a limited amount of lactic acid, which nurtures sperm as they make their way to the uterus.

When a woman climaxes, she does not ejaculate in the same way a man does. As her arousal increases, the flow of lubricating fluid increases. During climax, the muscles of the inner walls of the vagina ripple and contract, the intensity depending on the strength of these muscles. This pushes lubricant out of the vagina, something creating the appearance of ejaculation.

You can encourage your lover to strengthen her vaginal muscles by clenching and releasing them. They are the same muscles that a woman uses when she tries to stop urinating. Once these muscle are strengthened, just the act of rhythmically exercising her vagina will turn her on.

Don't TRY this (handwritten margin note)

The G-Spot

Even the doctors who discovered the G-spot aren't exactly sure where it is. It's somewhere on the front, inside the wall of the vagina. Good luck.

If you go searching for your lover's G-spot, you'll have to ask her how it feels as you rub certain spots. It's too analytical to be the most romantic experience you'll ever have. You'll have to think of it as a treasure hunt. Add a large dose of humor and you'll probably have a good time even if you never find it.

Breasts

Breasts are not technically part of the female genitalia, but they certainly are sensual zones.

Almost every woman has some reservation about the beauty of her breasts. They are too small, too big, too droopy... A good lover will assure his woman that her breasts are *perfect*, enticing, attractive, etc. It is not your business, and never will be any of your business, whether a woman should enlarge or reduce the size of her breasts. You could walk out of her life tomorrow, but her breasts will always be with her.

You should also know that most women's breast are not

exactly alike. One will be slightly larger than the other, or a slightly different shape.

When you fondle or kiss or suck on your lover's breasts, pay attention to her reactions. For some women, it is an extremely erotic sensation, akin to touching the clitoris. For other women, it's like rubbing on her elbow. Really.

Breasts don't respond well to squeezing, pressing, or pounding. Only a few women will enjoy having their breasts handled roughly, tugged, or bitten. For others, this sort of handling will kill the mood more quickly than anything. Just remember to watch *her*. Don't get carried away in your own enjoyment until you've made sure she's enjoying it, too.

Menstruation

This is nothing wrong with having sex while your lover is menstruating. The menstrual flow is not pure blood, but is mixed with the normal lubricant fluids present in the vagina. It's a perfectly natural function, and you will be much closer to your goal if you accept every aspect of your lover's body.

Some women actually feel more excited at this time of the month. Indeed, the muscle contractions during intercourse and climax can ease cramping.

Put down a towel if you're worried about the sheets. And have some slippery fun!

6 | *The Male Body*

Now you know a little more about the functions of the female body—but you also need to understand the mechanics of your own body. Your lover would also benefit from knowing this.

Semen

Semen is the viscous liquid, made up primarily of proteins, that is secreted through the urethra during arousal and final ejaculation. It also contains sperm, which are manufactured in each testis.

Seminal fluid can seep out of the penis once you have been aroused. This is very important to remember, because you can impregnate your lover without even climaxing.

Your Penis

The penis is mostly a shaft of spongy tissue that fills up with blood when a man is sexually aroused. The plumlike head of the penis or glans is particularly full of hypersensitive nerve endings.

Aside from slight variations, your lover won't be able to see much difference between your penis and her memory of another man's. The shape is pretty basic and without a comparison nearby, it's honestly very difficult to see what difference an inch makes. The average erect penis is about six inches long.

When you're making love, of course, the better your penis fits a woman's vagina, the more pleasure you both will have.

But the problems caused by a penis that is too large for a woman are worse than those caused by one that is small.

The other main concern about the penis is usually the quality and duration of your erection. Your erection is not solely dependent on the mechanisms of your penis—it ultimately rests on your mental and emotional states. The three main erection problems are listed below.

Premature Ejaculation

or You made a funny move

There is no time limit that defines premature ejaculation. *3 sec.* You are prematurely ejaculating if you *usually* climax before your lover can have an orgasm. Though it's not necessary every time, your lover won't be very pleased if she's never given enough of a chance to have an orgasm.

If your lover usually has no problem with orgasm, it's up to you to work on holding off. It's possible that you simply need to touch your lover more when you don't intend to have sex. Give her hugs and massages. Cuddle with her. That way, you won't want to climax simply from touching her.

Usually it just takes practice and training to keep yourself from ejaculating prematurely. Perhaps all you have to do is change your ideas about sex and decide not to climax as quickly. You could masturbate about an hour before you have intercourse. Or you could learn control by masturbating almost to climax—then stopping until you are under control—then continuing until you almost climax, then stopping again. You can strengthen the muscles that control ejaculation just as your lover can strengthen the muscles of her vagina. It's the same muscles that can stop the flow of urine. You could also wear a condom, which desensitizes your penis. There are plenty of options. Try a few.

Interrupted Intercourse

What do you do if you are making love and suddenly your erection starts to fade? If you're like most men, you tense up and try to keep on going, manipulating your penis inside your lover if you have to.

Don't worry about it. Most women understand that your erection is not completely voluntary, and absolutely anything can interfere. And this doesn't just happen to men.

Every woman has experienced a time during sex when she suddenly, inexplicably turns off. It could be an intrusive sound, or a sudden thought, or a painful movement. But women are able to bluff their way through whereas men cannot, and your lover knows this.

So don't try. Believe me, you aren't fooling anyone. Instead of ignoring it or feeling ashamed, be honest with your lover. Inevitably, her first thought will be that she's done something wrong or isn't attractive enough. She'll appreciate any explanation you have—whether it's because you've had too much to drink or you're not able to concentrate for whatever reason—much, much more than silence.

Alcohol, though it may make a man feel amorous, almost always interferes with a firm erection. Narcotics and tranquilizers do the same thing.

If you persistently are unable to maintain an erection, you should visit a doctor. There could be a physical reason for your problem.

Impotence

You shouldn't be concerned about occasional impotence. It's just one of the natural consequences of such a complex act, dependent on both physical and mental factors.

If the problem becomes chronic, the important thing is to find out why your are impotent. It could be simple anxiety about something in your sexual life or your relationship with your lover. It could be stress, fatigue, or outside pressures from family or job. It could be rooted in your attitudes about sex. It could be a health problem.

It is up to you to explore the possible reasons. You can't ignore what's happening and simply hope it will go away. Talk to your lover about it. She should know you pretty well. Talk to friends and family. See your doctor.

If you cover all possibilities, and are honestly at a loss for the reason, then there is still something you can do. A little home sex therapy. You and your lover should agree that there will be no intercourse for four weeks. That has to be the rule, and you both have to stick to it even if you do get a good erection. You should both cuddle and fondle one another, including your penis—even if it doesn't respond. Help her reach climax, with cunnilingus or masturbation. You'll find there are plenty of fun ways to have sex that don't rely on your penis. Usually all it takes for you to keep an erection is knowing that everything isn't dependent on it.

7 | *Appearance*

For women, the two basic factors of a man's appearance are: "Is he reasonably fit?" and "Is he clean?"

I'm sure you're aware that you can enjoy sex much more if you're in good shape. You're not going to be able to enjoy your orgasms as much if you're perspiring and completely out of breath the whole time.

But much more important to your lover than how fast you can run a mile is your personal cleanliness. Good hygiene is essential.

Grooming

It seems unnecessary to mention anything to do with personal cleanliness in this day and age. But unlike women, men are not conditioned by society or their peers to think their smell or grimy hands are of any importance. Women consider these things important. They ask themselves: Which deodorant works best? Should I douche or use a hygiene spray? Is my hair as clean as it could be? How is my makeup?

A woman is sensitized to these things, and will notice if her lover is not careful about his grooming. You may have to go above and beyond what you consider to be adequate grooming to reach the standard that your lover maintains. But few things can turn a woman off faster than bad breath, strong body odor, dirty hands, smelly feet or genitals. Beard stubble can be downright *painful*. It's not something you can ignore if you want to drive your woman wild.

Physique

In general, men place more importance on the appearance of their lovers than women do.

Your character will do more to further a relationship with your lover than your physical appearance. Even if you aren't the greatest looking man, any "flaws" will be greatly overshadowed by your wonderful self-confidence. Honesty, generosity, sensitivity, sense of humor, intelligence, imagination, courage, compassion, and confidence are what a woman considers desirable in a man.

And contrary to a popular male myth, your gym is not the key to driving your woman wild in bed. In fact, if you are addicted to exercise, you had better find a lover who is addicted, too. If your lover is not an exercise buff, it won't be high on her list of things to admire. She could even resent the time you spend working out.

To be in "good shape" for making love, all you need is a normal, healthy outdoor life involving physical activities such as team sports, biking, hiking, running, or swimming.

Her Physique

Many women wish men cared as much about a woman's character and intelligence as they do about her appearance. But it's also true that women have been raised basing a large part of their self-worth on their appearance. This contradiction remains unresolved in many women. It's something you have to take into account.

Women like to be praised—after all, they put extra effort into looking good. If you don't compliment your lover, she'll notice it and tensions will rise.

One quick way to alienate your lover is to tell her that she's fat or flabby or needs to dye her hair or wear more makeup. Your lover knows exactly what she looks like, better than you do. Make sure you have a solid relationship with your lover before your criticize her appearance. Always be complimentary before and *after* offering any advice on possible changes to make.

8 | *Contraception*

Worst case scenario: Your lover gets pregnant. Do you really want to deal with that? If you don't, you'd better take your share of responsibility for contraception.

Talking about contraception used to be a tougher problem than it is today. The difficulty of asking the question "Are you protected?" in the midst of a sexual encounter with a new lover seemed to stymie some men.

But in this day of AIDS, that question has become almost irrelevant. You should always wear a condom with your lover unless you are in a monogamous relationship with her. There's an estimated half-million undiagnosed cases of AIDS in America right now. This is not something you want to gamble with.

If you are in a monogamous relationship with your partner, and you both check negative for HIV, then there are methods of contraception other than the condom. Even today there still are some men who are uncomfortable discussing contraception because it doesn't fit the "mood" of sex. That is the most irresponsible and selfish attitude a man can take, and your lover will inevitably think the same thing.

Discussing contraception is not an offensive topic to women, nor will she take it as an invasion of privacy. After all, you are engaging in the most intimate activity that's possible between two people. And your choice of contraception will inevitably have an effect on your sexual relationship. You owe it to yourselves to talk about it together.

Condoms

The condom is often the contraception of choice in the AIDS era. Take time to find a brand of condoms with which you are comfortable. Some brands are thinner than others; some are lubricated with powder and jelly. You can get different colors, different textures, and even different sizes.

One type of condom you should know about is the lamb's skin condom. It is made from a part of the lamb's intestine. Lamb's skin condoms can be almost three times as expensive as the latex condoms, but they are natural and super-sensitive. But because they are made of natural material, there is some doubt about their ability to stop the AIDS virus. (For more on condoms, see the chapter on AIDS, page 31.)

The Pill

For many women, this is the preferred method of contraception. If your lover is on the Pill, she takes one every day. (The pills that fall on the days she is having her period are placebos or blanks, just to keep her in the habit.)

Contraceptive pills contain hormones that simulate pregnancy, preventing the woman from ovulating. The negative side effects can include weight gain, tender breasts, headaches, nausea; or worse, blood clotting and strokes. Her body may also have more difficulty producing vaginal lubrication.

The positive side effects can include reduced cramping, reduced menstrual flow, and reduced hormonal fluctuation—better known as PMS (premenstrual syndrome).

Some women don't like what the Pill does to their body. You should never pressure your lover to take the Pill because you think it will be easier or more convenient for you; it's your lover's decision.

Diaphragm

This is a stiff rubber ring, anywhere from two to three inches across, with a flexible rubber dome. It fits over the cervix and prevents sperm from entering the uterus. A spermicidal cream or gel must be used with the diaphragm so that it forms a seal when resting against the cervix.

The diaphragm should not be removed until at least six hours after intercourse. A fresh application of spermicide must be applied to the inside of the diaphragm before the next intercourse. As you can see, both hygienic concerns and the need to use fresh spermicide make it impossible for your lover to always wear her diaphragm just to be prepared for sex.

Cervical caps are simply smaller versions of the diaphragm. It's important that cervical caps are fitted correctly, since they adhere with a sort of suction directly to the cervix. Usually, spermicides aren't used with cervical caps, so they aren't as messy as diaphragms. However, cervical caps are more difficult to insert and remove.

If you can feel your lover's diaphragm or cervical cap, *tell her.* It could be that it has slipped from position and is no longer protecting her. You'll be the first to know, not her.

IUD

IUD is short for intrauterine device. This method involves the insertion of a small copper or plastic device through the opening of the cervix into the uterus (which must be done by a physician). It can be, among others, shaped in a coil or a T. It prevents a fertilized egg from embedding in the lining of the uterus.

The problems of IUD's involve penetration of the walls of the uterus or infection caused by the device. And, occasionally, a man's penis comes in contact with the small string attached to the IUD that sticks through the cervix. You'll know it when it happens.

Withdrawal

Risky business. Sperm leaks from the penis before a man actually ejaculates. Even the tiniest drop can impregnate a woman.

Also, you'll be thinking so much about controlling your ejaculation and pulling out in time that both you and your lover won't be able to fully enjoy the experience. You want to lose yourself when you have intercourse, not be calculating how long you can last before you have to withdraw.

Rhythm Method

This method involves having sex only on certain days of the month, when the woman is not fertile. Some women use a rather sophisticated combination of temperature readings and observation of the lubricant fluid coming from the cervix. Others simply estimate when their ovulation will occur according to the calendar—approximately fourteen days after the start of her last period.

Statistics show that users of this method bear more children than users of other methods.

9 | *AIDS*

Because of AIDS, sex has unfortunately become associated with both death and disease. The only way to ensure that your sexual experience is rewarding and pleasurable is by dealing with this issue in a positive way.

How Do You Get AIDS?

You owe it to yourself to learn the truth about AIDS. Anyone can get AIDS. It's not enough to avoid "high-risk groups"—bisexuals, homosexuals, and IV drug users. AIDS has been spread to every segment of the society, both male and female.

Technically speaking, the AIDS virus is hard to transmit. Casual contact—including toilet seats, doorknobs, touching, sweat, shaking hands, and sneezing—has been ruled out as a means of transmission.

AIDS is transmitted during the exchange of body fluids. The virus has been found in blood, semen, vaginal lubricant, urine, breast milk, saliva, and tears. Usually, your skin is enough to stop the virus from entering. But if any of these fluids come in contact with one of your bodily fluids, the virus has direct access into your body and can therefore be transmitted.

Though minute amounts of the AIDS virus have been found in saliva, kissing is not considered a risk factor in the transmission of AIDS. There has never been a recorded

31

instance of someone acquiring AIDS this way. If you are still concerned, then don't go in for the big, deep, sloppy kinds of kisses.

The high-risk fluids are blood and semen, and, to a lesser degree, vaginal lubricant. If your skin is broken in any way (on the rest of your body as well as your genitals), it can become an entrance for the AIDS virus.

It is easier to pass AIDS during anal sex because the inner lining of the anus is more delicate than the thick padding in the vagina. However, tiny tears are also made in the lining of the vagina during intercourse. This is a direct path to the bloodstream for the AIDS virus. The same goes for you. If your penis is chafed or the skin has been broken in any way, the virus has direct access to your bloodstream.

Experts recommend that you don't have sex that is coarse or forceful. And avoid inserting large objects into the vagina or anus.

Condoms

Use a condom. Pure and simple.

Some men say that it destroys the sensation and ruins their timing. These men aren't trying hard enough to find a condom that works for them.

You have to stop looking at condoms as a necessary but unpleasant part of your sexual encounters. The correct condom for you can mean the difference between lousy sex and outrageous sex.

For some men who ejaculate too quickly, a condom can help slow them down to enjoy the experience. Some men like the lubricated condoms—they're so slippery, sensationally wet! Other men liked the ribbed to stippled condoms for the extra stimulation they provide. There are also colored condoms and flavored condoms for oral sex.

If you are unhappy because of a dulling in your sexual

sensation, then buy thinner condoms! There are many different brands on the market. Keep in mind that some aren't guaranteed by the FDA to be as protective as the thicker latex condoms, but you still have a wide range from which to choose. And new products go on the market every day.

You owe it to yourself to try out different types of condoms to find the best one for you. After all, you don't go into a car dealership, gesture blindly to the first car you see, and say, "I'll take that one."

Sex is too important for you to be shy about this. Nowadays, the word condom is on everyone's lips—from twelve-year-olds to eighty-year-olds. You're doing the responsible thing, so hold your head high and request in a dignified tone, "Yes, the twelve pack, please."

What Do Women Think of Condoms?

For many women, using condoms for sexual intercourse has several nice side effects. Condoms are the easiest, healthiest contraceptive method available, and they prevent the transmission of sexual diseases.

Condoms also make sex more hygienic for women, especially if they engage in intercourse fairly often. The vagina isn't as easy to wash as your penis. And douching is harmful and irritating to the lining of the vagina if it is done too frequently.

If your lover wants you to use a condom, it is not your place to refuse. Your reasons are invariable selfish. Hers are based on health and hygiene. Even if you prevail, and the condom isn't used, your lover won't be entirely "with you" during intercourse. Part of her mind will be on that little bit of rubber lying on the ground, wondering why you don't care enough about her to use it. You'll never drive your lover wild in bed that way.

Tips on Using Condoms

Supply

Always have a condom with you. Don't worry that a new lover will think you're a sex-crazed maniac. She'll think you're a responsible man, and may even have her own condom supply in her purse.

Condoms have a tendency to dry out, especially if heated. If your condom feels flaky or stiff, then don't use it. Most manufacturers recommend not using a condom if it's more than two years old.

Bringing Up the Subject

You may be worried that bringing up the subject of condoms will destroy the mood. This isn't true. In fact, it isn't something that should be a big production. If you use condoms to practice safe sex, it's not a question you have to ask, like "Are you using birth control?" It's much easier than that. When you are getting close to penetration, simply pull the condom out, smile into her eyes as if you can't wait for what's next, and proceed to put it on.

Application

When you put the condom on, make it a sensual experience. Don't roll to one side of the bed, hunch over, and furtively slip it on. This ruins the mood. You both know the condom is going on, so what is there to hide? Make it an event. Display your erection. Stroke yourself. You can put your lover's hand on your penis and guide her in rolling it on. Always maintain some kind of contact with your lover, leaning against her or touching her with one hand.

Many women love to watch a man put a condom on. It's a chance for them to see their lover's erection, and the anticipation of having to pause for a moment only increases their desire.

Lubricants

Don't use oil-based lubricants when you're using a condom. They will make the condom disintegrate. This includes Vaseline and other petroleum jellys. Stick to water-soluble lubricants such as KY Jelly.

Removal

Like the application of a condom, the removal doesn't have to be an embarrassing event either. You probably won't want help with this, since your penis is sensitive. But again, don't run or roll away. To be a good lover, you have to be open about all the intimate details involved in the sexual experience. Your lover will appreciate it, and you both will gain more confidence with each other.

AIDS Testings

There is a blood test you can take that detects the antibodies which indicate you have been exposed to AIDS. You have to wait at least three months after your last sexual contact (or maintain a *strictly* monogamous relationship, in which both partners are tested). It takes time for your body to form the antibodies after exposure. Some people don't develop the antibodies until a year after exposure.

Some people are afraid to take the AIDS test. They think they would rather live with the fear than know the truth. But if fear of AIDS is affecting your life—you have intense flashes of dread and self-loathing, or you panic when you get sick—then take the test. There are things you can do to live healthily and happily even if you have the virus. It's better than the pervasive damage that fear can do to your life.

It's good to take an AIDS test before you get married. You're committing to a monogamous long-term relationship, so you should know each other's state of health. If one of you does have the antibodies, this doesn't necessarily mean that

AIDS will follow. It does mean that precautions should be taken when you have sex to prevent the uninfected partner from contracting the virus as well.

If you think you were exposed to the AIDS virus or you are in a "high-risk" group, you should take the AIDS test. You have a responsibility to not pass the virus on to your sexual partners.

Taking the AIDS test is not in itself a way to practice safe sex. You must always use a condom because your next partner might be infected. Just one unprotected contact can pass the AIDS virus.

Only you are responsible for your own health. There was an advertisement in the late eighties about AIDS that asked, "Is it worth dying for?" Ask yourself that question. Don't risk your future because you're embarrassed about protecting yourself, or you don't want to ruin the mood, or sex feels better without a condom. It's too big a gamble, and honestly, a few minutes of ecstasy is not worth your life.

It's easy, sitting here reading this book, to decide that you will always protect yourself. In the heat of the moment, however, you may not be so rational. Be prepared before you get into a sexual encounter. That means, buy condoms and always have them with you.

10 | *Massage*

Massage is an excellent way to both relax your lover and get to know her body. There are many different types of massage, from that found in the *Kama Sutra* to modern shiatsu. But sexual massage is a free-form art, which should be adapted to each situation and person.

Sexual massage can also be an easy bridge between casual contact and sexual intercourse. Whether it's an upright rub, with your lover sitting or standing, or a full-out affair with her naked and stretched out on your bed, massage is a nonthreatening sexual way to touch.

Remember, like anything else, massage is a learned skill. You have to do it to get better at it. And while you are doing it, listen to the feedback your lover gives you. If she winces or tenses, then you are pressing or rubbing too hard. Contrary to popular belief, a massage shouldn't hurt—especially a sexual massage. The idea here is to smooth and relax, not to give her a therapeutic workout of her muscles.

Manipulation

There are three basic methods of massage:

Stroking, with the palm or fingers of your hand. This can be done lightly or firmly, in short or long strokes. Stroking relaxes muscles and improves circulation to the small surface blood vessels. It is also thought to increase the flow of blood toward the heart.

Pressing, which includes kneading and squeezing. Pressing is usually targeted at particular muscles and joints.

Remember to keep your fingers stiffened and slanted when pressing. Reserve the tips of your fingers for joints and the large muscles of her back.

Percussion, in which the sides of the hands are used to strike the skin. This can be done rapidly or slowly, in varying degrees of strength. Percussions improves circulation.

Back Massage

A back massage can be anything from a quick rub at your coffee machine, to a sensual encounter complete with soft lights, music, and oil. Explore the full range of back massage with your lover.

Casual Rub

A casual rub is one that is done fully dressed. This kind of massage should be given freely with no sexual overtones attached. Your lover will interpret your brief massage as a desire for her to feel good, and she will appreciate your caring. Don't defeat your purpose by pressing this contact to a sexual encounter.

With the casual rub, don't get too involved. Target the muscles in her shoulders, neck, and upper back. Squeeze the top of her shoulders with your entire palm, pointing your stiffened fingers toward her neck and pressing your thumb and pinky together. Use your thumbs to rub the long, flat muscles between her shoulder blades and along her spine. Gently rub her neck up into her hair, putting your thumb on one side and fingers on the other—but remember to use your whole palm, not just the tips of your fingers, until you reach her skull. Against her skull you can use the tips of your fingers, rubbing hard in a circular motion. She should melt right under your hands. Restrain yourself, and finish off with a warm hug.

You can also use the casual rub to work into foreplay, but

make sure it doesn't always lead to sex. If this is the first time with your lover, make sure you've already given her a massage that didn't lead to sex.

It's best to work into foreplay via massage if you are both sitting down side by side, with your lover half turned away from you. You can suggest a massage quite casually—say that she looks tired or tense, and that you can fix that problem. Concentrate on relaxing her—don't feel her up in a sexual way or start sighing or moaning. Once you've given her a good rub, she'll be very relaxed and won't resist if you begin kissing the back of her neck and hugging her from behind. She'll turn to kiss you, or you can pull her across your lap, brushing her hair from her face as you look down at her. It will drive your lover wild when you hold her this way. No

Back Rub

Your lover should be lying down, so you can apply pressure as well as squeezing and stroking. Start from her side, kneeling or standing near her hips rather than straddling them. It's also good to use a lotion or oil—and, if you can, use her brand since that is the kind she likes. Women are very sensitive to what they put on their skin; how it feels as well as how it smells.

Rub her upper back and neck first, since this is the obvious tension-collecting spot. Press your palms against her back—but not too hard!—and rub in small circles. Follow the contours of her body and you'll feel the muscles beneath her skin that you can press and knead. And don't forget her neck up into her hair; it's a very relaxing sensation.

After giving her a thorough rub on her upper back, then work your way down. Again, follow the contours of her body. Just because it's a back massage, don't stick to the top of her back—encircle her waist with your hands, stroking her skin up to her chest and back down to her hips. Pay special attention to the soft area above her buttocks and below her waist. Rub this gently with your thumbs as your fingers encircle her hips. Don't press too hard on her lower back.

It's not as important as her back, but you can also rub her buttocks. The muscle is deeply buried under a layer of fat, so don't squeeze her buttocks, or you'll just hurt and irritate her. Press your stiffened fingers into her skin, firmly stroking upward from the tops of her thighs. Use long strokes. The muscles in her thighs are closer to the skin and more receptive to massage. If you don't start at her thighs, the buttock rub will feel a little silly to her.

Full Body Massage

With a full body massage, you can and should touch every part of her body. The secret is to know how long to dwell on each part.

Always start with her back when you're giving your lover a full body massage. If you have your lover lie down naked and start with her toes, she'll simply tense up and won't enjoy the experience. Massaging her back will relax her quickly and the rest of her body can follow pleasurably.

From her thighs, move down her legs to her feet. When you rub her legs, don't just rub the backs. Put both your hands around her leg, massaging firmly with your palm and squeezing the base of your thumb toward your straightened fingers. Don't press your fingertips into her skin unless it's around a joint. Rub all the way down to her knee, paying special attention to the joint around her kneecap, then back up. Then do the other leg. From there, work down to her ankles, again being particularly firm around her joints, then back up and to the other leg. When you reach her ankles, grasp one in each hand and gently lift and pull. This will help loosen the muscles in her legs. Then do her feet.

When you move back up to do her arms, first rub her upper back for a little while. This is supposed to be a total process, not a systematic ticking off of the parts. You don't have to spend as much time on her arms as you did her with legs. The muscles aren't used as much and don't have the same sort of tension. When you reach her wrist, grasp it in one hand and brace your other hand against her shoulder, pulling gently. This will loosen the muscles in her arms better than anything. Then turn your attention to her hands (see below).

Finish off with another quick rub of her neck and head.

Frontal Massage

If you want to turn your lover over to massage her chest and stomach, it's important to know that even an experienced masseuse won't spend much time on the front of a woman as they do with a man. A woman's stomach is too delicate for firm massage. Most men tend to focus on the breasts anyway, which are next to useless to massage. The muscles around the breasts can benefit, but again, a woman is much more delicate than a man and her rib cage cannot take the sort of frontal massage a man's can.

Foot and Hand Massage

As with the casual rub, foot and hand massage can be done without any sexual connotations. It's an excellent way to touch your lover and give her attention.

Hands

Lotion is optional. Practice first on your own hands, or your won't understand the feelings that you are creating.

Hold her upturned hand with your fingers at the back and your thumb in her palm. Rub your thumb and fingers together very firmly in a circular motion against the pad right below her thumb—particularly in the fleshy part between her thumb and fingers. When you rub the rest of her palm with your thumb, rub up toward her fingers, and you can't go wrong.

You can also grasp her entire hand in yours, squeezing her thumb toward the other side of her palm. Start at the wrist, rubbing the joint and turning it in your hand, then work toward her fingertips, squeezing her fingers together in yours.

Place each finger in the second joint of your fingers, with your thumb on the inside. With a circular motion, rub your thumb and fingers back and forth as you work your hand to the very tip. Pull gently on her finger as you do this. Massage each finger once or twice.

Feet

The principles are the same as for hand massage. Your thumb should be against the sole of her foot, with your fingers massaging the top. Her heel is like the pad of her thumb. The arch of her foot is more delicate, like the rest of her palm, and should be massaged more gently. The upper pad and toes should be treated like fingers, with your hands pulling out to the tips. Her big toe can take a firmer touch than her little toes.

Massage her ankle, in the tender area between her ankle bone and above her heel. Rotate her foot, loosening the tension in her ankle.

As with a back rub, a good hand or foot massage will do more to relax your lover than almost anything else.

11 | *Kissing and Petting*

You didn't think you had anything to learn about kissing or petting, didn't you?

Well, you're wrong. Both kissing and petting (sexual touching) are very important parts of your sexual encounters. You have to master the basics before you'll be able to drive your woman wild in bed.

Kissing

Kissing is the first threshold of intimacy. If your lover is turned off by your kiss, then you'll never get her *into* bed, much less drive her wild.

Do's and Don'ts

Don't be rough or forceful when you kiss. Take your time and use your lips as if they were fingers, to touch and caress her lips and skin.

Don't keep your mouth tightly puckered. The attraction of your lips is their mobility and soft, sensual nature. On the other hand, don't open your mouth wide and plaster it over hers.

Don't make your kiss too wet. It's not sexy if she has to wipe her face afterward. This goes for kissing any part of her body, as well as mouth to mouth.

Lastly, don't concentrate on your tongue. A kiss is mostly lip contact. If you go at your lover as if you intend to penetrate her with your tongue, there's a good chance she'll be turned off. Your collection of tongue techniques will make her feel as if there's a fish flopping around in her mouth. Always use your tongue gently on your lover.

Body Kissing

Kissing your lover's neck can be very erotic. That's kissing—not sucking. Not many people enjoy receiving a hickey or carrying it around as a testimony of last night's sex.

Gently kiss and trail your tongue under her chin and around her neck to under her ear. This is also a good way to get your lips from her mouth down to her breasts.

When it comes to ears, you should go slowly to make sure your lover likes it. For some women, it's the most uncomfortable, unsexy thing in the world to have a wet tongue in her ear. Don't ruin the mood by not paying attention to your lover's reaction.

One area to kiss that is often neglected is your lover's hand. The hand and fingers are packed with nerves and are particularly receptive to a kiss. You can kiss her palm and inner wrist; gently lick or suck on her fingers; press the back of her hand against your lips. The beauty of hand kissing is it can be done at any time, and should be indulged in freely.

Other sensitive places to plant a kiss are the crook of your lover's arm, her stomach and navel, inside her thighs, the back of her knees and her feet, her bare shoulders....

Petting

Good petting isn't just aimed at the genitals. You've got a whole, big, beautiful body to play with. Petting can be done with your clothes on or off, and should be combined with kissing.

Clothed

There is a certain titillation in touching your lover sexually while you are both still dressed. And there is no better prelude to a sexual encounter.

Don't zero in on your lover's breasts or genitals; petting should involve a slow, nonagressive technique. Run your hands over her body, feeling every curve and mound through her clothes. It will make her feel like she isn't wearing any clothes at all.

Full body contact is important, too, either lying down or standing up. Some people simply call this cuddling. You and your lover may actually be more comfortable with your clothes on. It's an easy way to get used to how your bodies feel together.

Naked

This is everything that clothed petting is, and more.

Take time to explore your lover's body with your hands. Firmly run your palms down her sides. Rub her buttocks and thighs with an upward, circular motion. Stroke her hair and trace the lines of her face. If you adore your lover's body, she'll adore you.

An Alternative to Intercourse

There is nothing stopping you from rubbing and touching each other until you climax. Petting is nonthreatening and more emotion-based than actual intercourse—and neither one of you has to worry about disease or contraception. Unfortunately, many men don't like to climax during a petting session. It might be the sticky spot on their shorts, or they might feel it's not really sex. Rest assured, it is.

In fact, for many women, petting can be even better than intercourse. It's not easy for men to understand, but women don't always have to climax to be sexually satisfied. It's the closeness and constant touching that your lover will go wild for.

It's very important for you to remember this. Intercourse should not be the primary goal of every sexual encounter. If you always end up with intercourse, eventually there will be no suspense in your sexual relationship. Petting is an exciting alternative that your lover will appreciate deeply.

12 | *Masturbation*

Masturbation is a necessary part of your sexual life. There are two good reasons to masturbate—to give yourself erotic pleasure, and to help you discover more about your own sexual responses. Like men, almost all women masturbate to some degree or another. Most people are reserved about admitting it, but unless a person masturbates, they will never be able to fully know what their own sexual likes and dislikes are.

One way to drive your lover wild in bed is by helping her expand her sexuality as much as possible. Encourage your lover to masturbate. It is simply not true that strongly stimulating a woman's clitoris will make her dependent on this in order to climax. Indeed, the more a woman masturbates, the more she learns about her own body—which, in turn, helps her learn how to reach climax better. You can then use this knowledge during intercourse with you.

Masturbating with Your Partner

Since masturbation is such a personal experience, some people are reluctant about touching themselves in front of their partner. Yet, masturbating in front of each other can greatly enhance your intimacy, and once you are comfortable, it can open an enormous range of sexual interaction.

Masturbation is an excellent alternative to intercourse, and can be as fully shared and explored with your lover as different positions or sexual acts. Your lover will learn about

47

your sexual responses by watching you masturbate, just as you will be better able to understand hers.

And keep in mind, it is not necessary to masturbate to climax—self-stimulation can occur at any point during sex and should be encouraged in both men and women.

13 | *Oral Sex*

Your mouth is an extremely sensitive organ. With it you are able to taste, touch, and smell your lover's body. In fact, your mouth is a lot like your genitals—rich in nerve endings and very receptive to stimulation. It makes sense to bring your mouth and genitals together.

Many people are put off by the closeness between the sex organs and the organs of excretion. Women know that the penis is used for urinating as well as sex, and some may be concerned that it is contaminated by urine. Men usually have the idea that there's someplace in a woman's crotch that urine comes from, perhaps even contaminating the whole area.

With ordinary hygiene, the sex organs can be as germ-free and clean-smelling as any other part of the body. In fact, the mouth usually contains a great many more germs than the penis or vulva. Sexual secretions, such as sperm and the lubricating fluids from the vagina, are antiseptic and harmless protein substances.

If you or your lover are still worried about cleanliness, then take a shower together! It's a great method of foreplay, and you won't have a question in your mind that your lover is squeaky clean.

After cleanliness, it's usually just a lack of knowledge about each other's genitals that keeps people from enjoying oral sex. Learn all you can, and enjoy the wide range of sensations available from oral sex.

Cunnilingus

Please do. You enjoy being on the receiving end of oral sex; your lover will, too.

The lubricating fluids have a distinctive smell and taste that varies in each woman. Since it is so closely associated with intercourse, many men are turned on by this scent. Other men aren't.

Without a doubt, if you want to drive your woman wild in bed, you have to accept every part of her body. If you don't like touching her genitals, much less kissing her there, you'll never be a great lover. And if you only come near her genitals to penetrate her, your lover will assume you're repelled by this part of her body. No woman likes that. You won't drive her wild, you'll drive her away.

On the other hand, if it's your lover who is reluctant to have you perform cunnilingus, then all you need to do is talk to her about it. Tell her how much you want to please her, and that you would love to kiss every part of her. If you're sincere, you won't have any problems. Once you start, she'll wonder why she ever protested.

Technique

Just as a woman uses both her hands as well as her mouth during fellatio, a man should use his hands as well as his mouth during cunnilingus. The question is, how?

When a woman is aroused, any part of her vulva is sensitive, but if you don't make contact with the clitoris it will simply frustrate her.

One thing you should keep in mind: The clitoris is a very protected part of a woman's body and therefore is extremely sensitive. If you overstimulate the clitoris—rubbing too hard or too fast or too long—it will be painful for your lover.

Pay close attention to your lover's reactions while performing cunnilingus. That is the only way you'll be able to discover what is pleasurable for her.

Some things you can do are: Use your tongue on the clitoris, flicking it against the small hood. Use your lips to rub against the ridge of the clitoris, shaking your head back and forth. Gently suck on the small pea-shaped protuberance. Rub the entire mound with the palm of your hand in an upward, circular motion.

While doing this, use your fingers to gently stroke the lips of the vulva. If the vagina is lubricated, knit two fingers together and insert them. Rhythmically move them in and out, or simply explore the interior of the vagina with your fingers.

If you move your mouth to any other part of her vulva, gently rub a finger against her clitoris or mound as you do. You may have to push your hands against her thighs to keep them open, especially if she begins to climax.

Some women like to be touched on the bridge of flesh between the opening of the vagina and the anus. The anus itself is sensitive, with many nerve endings. Be alert to your lover's movements when you touch the area around a woman's anus. If she clenches her cheeks together or pulls away at all, then don't press it. Some women simply don't like to be touched there. On the other hand, if your lover presses toward you or lets out a moan of delight, then probe away. A good lover pays attention to the nonverbal signals, and if you are uncertain, then ask! Whisper, "Like that? Higher?" giving her two options. She won't want to say she doesn't like it, but if she doesn't, she'll respond "higher."

Fellatio

No woman can know what it feels like to have your penis stroked. Just as you must want to perform cunnilingus on your lover, a woman must want to perform fellatio in order to do it well.

She may be clumsy, just as you would be if you didn't know a woman's anatomy. Talk to her about your genitals.

Show her what feels good. Don't let her keep on doing something that isn't comfortable. You'll never have a better chance to gracefully adjust her technique than during the first couple of times she performs fellatio on you.

[handwritten: YEAH THAT'S RIGHT!]

Don't try to force your lover to take more of your penis in her mouth. A gag reflex is triggered when something is pushed against the back of the throat. If you want your fun abruptly broken off, with your lover coughing and choking all over you, you'll let her control the action.

[handwritten: AND IT GAVE A NASTY TASTE IN YOUR MOUTH]

Don't feel rejected if your lover doesn't swallow your semen. It's not like anything else, rather a gooey glob that some women have difficulty swallowing. As long as she doesn't shy away from putting your penis in her mouth and enjoys bringing your to climax this way, you've got nothing to complain about. But whatever you do, if your lover has swallowed your come, don't reject a kiss from her.

69

In this position, your head is near her crotch while hers is near yours. This can be accomplished by lying on your sides, facing each other. Or, one partner lies on his or her back while the other props him or herself over.

Some people are talented enough to be able to give oral sex while receiving it. Others think it's crazy to ruin such a wonderful feeling by trying to concentrate on something else at the same time. It's purely a personal decision, so pay attention to your lover's reaction when you start to swing around in a 69 position. If she doesn't actively encourage it, then stick with one-at-a-time methods.

14 | *Orgasm*

The most important thing you need to remember about your orgasm is to *forget* about it. Don't put so much emphasis on the climax. There's a whole, long, wet, and wonderful road between your first kiss and the end of your sexual encounter. Think of your orgasm as the cherry on top of an ice-cream sundae, or a banana split, or a ———. You fill in the blank—and enjoy it while you're filling it in.

As for *her* orgasm, don't turn it into a quest for the holy grail. Sometimes, your lover simply won't climax. It doesn't mean she didn't thoroughly enjoy having sex with you; remember, your lover invests more emotional weight on being intimate with you. The physical satisfaction is only half of the experience.

Simultaneous Orgasm

It's not necessary and it will get in the way of your enjoyment if you're always seeking a simultaneous orgasm as the object of intercourse. It's the entire experience that's important, not the destination.

You must be familiar with your lover's technique and rhythms to orchestrate a simultaneous orgasm, and even then it's not predictable. Usually, when a woman climaxes, the muscles contract in the vagina, and this helps bring a man to orgasm. It's a one-two punch, rather than one big bang.

If Your Lover Can't Reach Orgasm

There's nothing mysterious about orgasm. If your lover does not reach orgasm, her nerves simply aren't being stimulated enough. She needs to relax and learn about her own sexual responses.

Just as men learn to reach orgasm through masturbation, the easiest way for a woman to learn to reach orgasm is through masturbation. You should encourage any woman who has trouble climaxing to masturbate. Buy her a vibrator! Then let her experiment with it on her own. The best way for her to reach orgasm is to relax, and she may not be able to do that with you hanging over her while she's learning. Don't feel excluded—the best thing you can do for your sexual relationship is to encourage your lover to explore her own sexuality, at her own pace.

When you do have sex together, take time for longer and more intensive foreplay. This doesn't mean leaping for her clitoris and rubbing away briskly. Work up slowly to the more intimate aspects—after all, what you have here is relaxation problem. Stroke her skin and kiss her. Encourage her to touch you in the same way.

Only when you both are comfortable should you move on to more intensive foreplay. Your lover should stimulate her own sex organs. Have her show you what feels good. Spend some time arousing her, but don't insist on bringing her to climax every time. The pressure of your expectations will destroy any progress your lover may make.

For many women, sex begins in their heads and hearts, not their sex organs. If your lover has trouble having orgasm with you in *particular*, perhaps what is missing is the romance in your relationship (see Romance). Make it a point to touch your lover at times other than during sex. Make it a point to tell her how much you care about her.

Although women also enjoy sex because of the ecstasy of climax, they really do place equal importance on the closeness they receive during intercourse.

15 | *Intercourse Positions*

The key to mutually satisfying sexual intercourse is to be spontaneous. You have unlimited freedom to create a sexual encounter from a "quickie" to an evening-long seduction. Falling into a rut is the beginning of the end for your sexual relationship.

Don't just make love on the bed. Remember that hot scene in *The Postman Always Rings Twice* when they sweep the dishes off the table and have sex right there? That scene wouldn't be so hot if they had restrained themselves and walked to bed. Be inventive. Your sofa may be the perfect height for you to kneel beside it and penetrate your lover as she sits on the very edge. Tables and counters are great for her to lean over. That nice plushy rug may be the perfect spot to lay her down.

You should also vary the type of coital thrusting you do. There's the slow, steady circular thrust. There's the rapid-fire thrust. There's the rhythm that increases in tempo. Your lover can also set the rhythm. Don't just stick with one all the time, just as you don't want to always use the same position for intercourse.

Of the following intercourse positions, there are a hundred variations for each. You should feel free to experiment.

There's nothing stopping your from changing positions several times during intercourse, but beware of breaking the mood with elaborate manipulations. It must happen naturally. Don't try to impress your lover with how many ways you know to have intercourse. Under no circumstances does a woman want to feel as if she's being run through a catalog of positions. She'll start to wonder what she's done wrong in the last three positions that wasn't satisfying you. She definitely won't be relaxed, and she won't be able to climax.

The most important thing to remember about position is that it's a secondary concern. Your lover will find it far more important to be comfortable with you, feeling your arms around her, and listening to your whispered words of affection.

Missionary Position

You on top, facing your lover. This position is good for kissing and caressing as you have intercourse.

Missionary position usually refers to both partners stretched out on a horizontal surface, but it can also include your lover lying near the edge of the bed or couch while you kneel in front of her.

While lying stretched out on the bed, the main variables come in with the positioning of her legs. One way is to wrap her legs around your hips or upper thighs. This position does not necessarily mean you control the rhythm. However, it does restrict the movements of her hips, since she is holding on to you.

Another way is to pull one or both of your lover's legs forward, bracing them against your shoulders. This allows deeper penetration than the normal missionary position. However, the woman's hips are pinned against the bed, and thus cannot respond to your motions. If you want to be in control, this is a good position. But if you always want to have intercourse this way, you must make sure you get a lover who is aroused by being passive.

The ideal position, if you want to drive your woman wild, is for her to bend her knees slightly and brace her feet against the bed. This allows her to push against your thrust. In this position, you will be aware of the rhythm that she is seeking and will know if you are going too fast, too slow.

too evenly, or whatever. In this position, you can move together.

Reverse Missionary Position

Her on top, you on bottom. This usually refers to you lying stretched out on the bed, with her straddling your hips. Your lover can also place her feet beneath her, squatting over you, but it's usually more comfortable for her to kneel on her knees. Another way is for you to sit on a chair with your lover facing you in your lap.

You get to relax in this position and let your lover do more of the work. Even better, your hands are free to caress her. You may want to grip her waist or hips to help control the rhythm. You can also pull her chest down or push her up to change the angle of penetration.

Don't let old stereotypes keep you from enjoying this position. Sometimes your lover may have more energy than you, while you want to lie back and enjoy. Sometimes you may want to be free to caress her during intercourse.

Rear Entry

You both face the same way, with you behind your lover. You can both stand, with your lover leaning over slightly to aid in penetration. It can also be done with your lover on all fours with you kneeling behind her. More difficult is with both of you lying together on your sides, your lover in front and you curled around her. This allows deep penetration, but it's hard to get a good rhythm going with your hips, lying on the bed.

The rear entry offers you a different view of your lover. Since she can only see the wall, it is very important to caress her with your hands, even leaning over to hug her from behind. If you simply hold her hips, that can be exciting too, but it is inherently more impersonal.

Since this position is not as intimate as the first two, some women don't like it. In a woman's definitions of making love and having sex, this position is usually considered to be sex. In addition, since penetration is deeper, it can also be painful. Be aware of her reactions.

On the other hand, many women love the feeling of submission and raunchy fun implicit in this position. It is truly something that has to be tried to find out how exciting it can be. Since domination is implied on the part of the man, you are free to pursue this position a little more aggressively than you should with other positions or sexual enhancements. However, if your lover is truly repelled by this position, then you'll have to wait for a lover who is more receptive.

Other Variations

There are hundreds of positions for sex. Any of these basic positions can be varied by moving an arm or leg, as in the scissor position. You can stand face to face, with one of your lover's legs raised or propped up on the bed. You can kneel between your lover's legs, holding her hips up in your arms as her chest and head rest on the bed. Use pillows to brace her hips or chest higher. The variations are limited only by your imagination.

16 | *Where and When*

You should fit your sexual encounters to the ambience. If it's a "quickie" in the kitchen, there won't be a lot of romance going on. Under the fluorescent lights, it will be more like hot, raw sex. Or you can create a sensual ambience for a slow, erotic session by dimming the lights, using candles, or lighting a fire. Don't get in the habit of always doing the same thing just because it is familiar and comfortable. Sex should be exciting, and sometimes a change as small as going from light to dark can be enough to add an erotic spark to your sexual encounters.

Where

Your lover can get even more excitement from *where* you have sex than *how* you have sex. Keep it new and exciting, even if it means having intercourse in different rooms of your house or whispering how much she's turning you on while you're in a crowded room.

Sex is a sensual experience, and sensuality is heightened when your are using all your senses. You limit yourself when you limit the surroundings in which you make love. You'll never know how exciting it can be to have sex in a place that is unusual for you until you try it.

Anyplace in the world is a potential place to make love. It might turn out to be uncomfortable or hurried, but the sheer eroticism of having intercourse in a car, or outdoors, or in the bathroom at a party is worth every inconvenience. You wouldn't want to give up the comfort and privacy of your own bedroom, but if you seize the moment, you will have an experience that will be memorable.

You can either plan your sex in unusual places, or it can be spontaneous.

If you plan on having sex anywhere unusual, make sure you work it out completely beforehand. You don't want to be stopped after you've presented the plan to your lover and you've both gotten all excited. This will just cause frustration.

Your lover may be reluctant and afraid that you will be "caught." Don't push her into it, but don't hesitate to suggest making love when you see a good place or time to do it. Your lover may just need to accustom herself to the idea. Get her excited about it.

By consistently expressing your physical attraction to your lover, you will do a great deal to enhance your sexual relationship. If you reserve sex for special occasions or a certain place, you will be isolating it from the rest of your relationship. Never let sex become a routine if you want to drive your woman wild in bed.

When

It's not a good idea to always have sex at the same time of day every time.

Your body chemistry fluctuates throughout the course of the day, and your sexual experience will change along with it. Particularly with a new lover, you owe it to yourselves to experience sex at different times. Some people are unresponsive during certain parts of the day, while at other times they can hardly hold back. You need to get to know your lover's rhythms and preferences.

Many men take advantage of the morning erection (the pressure of urine in the bladder produces an erection). But many women find this to be an unromantic time of day.

Among other things, it is uncomfortable for a women to have sex with a full bladder. The pressure can even cause a urinary infection. If you want sex in the morning, pay attention to your lover's reaction. Suggest that she go to the bathroom, or you both can brush your teeth. Make it comfortable for her, and you'll both have a great time.

Afternoon sex can be quite wonderful, too. It can add a certain thrill to make love during a time you are normally hard at work.

Quickies can take place at any time, and should be encouraged. After all, that is what they are for. Try one in the evening before you go out together, while making breakfast on Sunday, or on your way out the door to work.

The most usual time to have sex is at night, just before going to sleep. The problem is that many people are simply too tired by then to create a really enjoyable sexual experience. Sex becomes routine. If you find yourself falling into this habit, make the effort to have your sexual encounter earlier in the evening.

Take time for sex, for trying new things. Put the spark back in your relationship that was almost lost due to poor timing and lack of spontaneity.

17 | *A Few Things to Keep in Mind*

Besides the Where and When of sex, covered in the last chapter, *how* you go about the sexual encounter with your lover is important, too. Talking, creative sex play, passionate rather than robotic intercourse, and basking in the *afterglow* (a particularly meaningful part of sex for women) are all important factors to consider when it comes to pleasing your partner.

Talking During Sex

It can be a turn-on for your lover to hear you murmur in her ear. But always set the tone of your conversation by hers. If she doesn't use dirty words, then you will be making a huge mistake by using gutter language with her in bed. That's one thing that can really make women feel like sex objects.

On the other hand, romantic comments, repeating her name, groaning or moaning, or saying yes or please are surefire ways to drive your woman wild. Men more often make the mistake of being unnaturally silent while having sex. Women are verbally attuned, and a murmured word of love or adoration will do more to increase her excitement than any fancy physical technique you may have picked up.

Length of Intercourse

You probably know that you won't be able to drive your woman wild in bed if just pop in and out, and climax without paying any attention to her emotions and sexual needs. But this doesn't mean your lover will be impressed by the length of time you can have intercourse before climaxing.

Do you need that to be repeated?

Only men are concerned with the length of their sexual performance. And if you do everything you can to draw it out, that's exactly how a woman will look at it—a performance. She'll be looking around for the dog and pony show that comes on next.

Just because women can have multiple orgasms doesn't mean that you have to make her climax a dozen times to be great in bed. Most women are satisfied with one real good one. Sometimes just being close is enough.

Sexual intercourse should be a mutual project. If you are thinking of your bills or your mother to keep from climaxing, that's not very complimentary to your lover. She wants you to be thinking only of *her*. If she's responding and having a good time, she'll wonder why you are holding back. And how can she climax if you aren't trying to?

The most complimentary thing you can do is to act as if you can't control yourself—she's so beautiful, it feels so good, you're in ecstasy!

Afterglow

For heaven's sake, when it's over, it's *not* over. Maintain some sort of contact, don't just roll away panting or jump out of the bed to wash yourself. This is downright offensive and will give your lover the feeling that you got what you wanted and aren't interested in her anymore.

And if you're complaining that you get sleepy and can't help it—you're *wrong*. The male desire for sleep after climax only lasts for a few minutes. If you fight your drowsiness right at the beginning, it will go away, leaving you feeling better than ever.

So, if you want an ongoing, satisfying sexual relationship with your lover, don't turn off once you've climaxed. Run your hand lightly over her skin. Gently kiss her or touch her hair. Simply hold hands or rest against each other. Look into her eyes. No matter what happened while you were having intercourse, she will think you are a great lover just for paying her this extra attention.

Afterglow is not just physical. Talk to your lover. You've just engaged in the most intimate contact possible—what's left to hide? Tell her things you would never bring up normally—desires, dreams, memories. You both are more tender at this time than any other. Take advantage of it and you'll drive your lover wild.

The First Time with Your Lover

Since sexual satisfaction is such an individual thing, it's common for two people to be awkward with each other the first few times they have intercourse. Personal rhythms are different, and each of you are accustomed to doing things a certain way based on past sexual encounters.

In order to drive your woman wild in bed, you must be aware of how she is reacting to what you say and do, and adjust accordingly. You must take into account her pleasure rather than concentrating on getting your own. If you do this with your lover right from the first, then your rewards will be greater than you can imagine.

Long-term Relationships

Are you being creative enough in your sex life? Or have you allowed it to become routine? Are you doing the same old things over and over?

In a long-term relationship, you can't expect the erotic freshness and thrill to remain as spine-tingling as it was in the first few weeks. But if you both work at keeping it alive, then there is no reason why you should drift apart physically, through tedium and lack of inspiration.

Also, it's good if you can inject a lightness and sense of play into your sexual relationship. If you put some humor along with the romance into your sex life, you'll go a long way toward increasing your mutual satisfaction.

Hopefully, you will be in a long-term relationship at one time or another. Searching for sexual excitement by moving from one lover to the next will inevitably end in failure for you. Your first excitement will always fade as you become familiar with your lover. Unless you can come to terms with that, you will never reach full sexual satisfaction because you will never progress beyond a certain level in your sexual experience.

18 | *Fantasies*

Fantasy has a large part to play in everyone's sex life. You can fantasize privately to control or stimulate your sexual responses, or you can reveal your innermost fantasies to your lover.

Many people can accept this sort of fantasizing, but they hesitate when it comes to acting out their fantasies. Don't eliminate that possibility from your sexual encounters—if done in an atmosphere of trust and mutual esteem, acting out your fantasies can be an exciting experience.

Private Fantasies

There's no need to worry that you or your lover are not being "true" to one another, or that there's something wrong with your relationship if you fantasize. Fantasizing is a healthy part of your sexuality. The more aroused and excited you are, the more passionate and adventurous you'll be.

Sharing Fantasies

Sharing your fantasies with your lover can provide fun, variety, and excitement, and at the same time create greater intimacy in your sexual relationship. Trust is very important in this case, so if either one of you isn't comfortable, then wait until you know one another better.

Acting Out Fantasies

Good communication is necessary before you can act out a fantasy. It's really a role-playing game, with rules you set to define your roles before your begin. It can be as mild as assigning one of you to be the aggressor in seducing the other. Or you can pick different personalities, and see what happens when you come together. Or you can turn your fantasy into a full-fledged production, complete with costumes and lines.

Fantasies are a good way to include a wider range of sex acts in your encounters than if you simply suggested them out of the blue. If you've always wanted to tie up your lover, a nonthreatening way to suggest this is by telling her about your fantasy of bondage. If she is receptive and turned on by your fantasy, then, later, you can ask her if she wants to enact it with you.

Remember, not all fantasies are meant to be acted out. If your lover is uncomfortable with the idea, then it's best to drop it. Acting out your fantasies should be a fun, intriguing experience, not something that causes tension between you and your lover.

YES. I WILL BE ROCK STUDLY AND YOU WILL BE PRICILLA. YOU WILL RECEIVE!

19 | *Sex and Your Bathroom*

Many women enjoy the wide range of sexual activities that can take place in the bathroom.

Like massage, taking a shower or bath is a good way to get comfortable with your lover and accustomed to her body. The immediate pressure of sex is submerged in the purpose of getting clean.

Sex in the bathroom is usually more erotic than romantic. So keep it lighthearted until passion takes over.

Shower

Make sure the water temperature is good for both of you. One man's warm is another woman's scalding.

Soap is great because it eases the friction of skin on skin. Don't use harsh, deodorant soap. But clear glycerine soap, or soap made with lanoline, vitamin E, and cocoa butter.

When you get into the shower together, restrain yourself from leaping for her breasts or genitals. Offer to wash her back. Rub shampoo into her hair and rinse it for her. Massage and wash her feet. Make it a total body experience.

When you have intercourse in the shower, be very careful that you don't slip. Slow, languorous, sensual intercourse is the key to bathroom sex, or you'll end up at the hospital instead of snuggled together in bed. The shower or bathtub is not the place to be rough or wild.

Bathtub

Depending on the size of your tub, it can be fun to share a bath together. Light some candles, listen to music, and relax in the warm water together. You can put a couple of drops of her perfume in the water or oil beads or even bubble bath. This should be a sensual, comfortable experience.

Quickies

The bathroom is also a good place for a quickie, whether it's in someone else's bathroom or your own. The edge of the tub, the toilet seat, and the plushy rug are all good places for sex. And don't forget the sink—it's the perfect height for your lover to brace herself against as you penetrate her from behind.

20 | *Anal Eroticism*

This includes the erotic stimulation of the anus, either by fingers, sex toys, or your penis.

Anal Stimulation

Gentle stimulation of the anus is a common way of adding to sexual excitement. The anus itself is sensitive, with many nerve endings. Be alert to your lover's movements, however, when you touch the area around the anus. ~~Some women simply don't like to be touched there.~~ On the other hand, if your lover presses toward you or lets out a moan of delight, then go right ahead.

There's no limit to the way you can stimulate the anus. You can stroke or tickle the puckered ridges of the anus itself. Run your fingers up the crack. Massage the buttocks and upper thighs. Rub the bridge of flesh between the anus and vagina. Some women (and men) like to have a finger A Bfrl'c inserted into their anus during sex.

You can also use a vibrator or dildo to stimulate your lover's anus. As with anal intercourse, this has to be done very carefully.

Anal Intercourse

Submit

Anal intercourse is something both partners have to ~~want~~ to do before it can be successful. A lot of men like to perform anal intercourse, because the rectum is much tighter than the vagina, and they can get more powerful stimulation more quickly. Since the muscles in the anus are so strong, it will be impossible to penetrate your lover without causing both pain and damage if she doesn't like what's happening. Your lover must be relaxed. *the BFHC*

Lubricant will ease the insertion of your penis. *the* At first, go slow and steady until her muscles have fully relaxed and your lover realizes that you aren't going to hurt her. *him*

Positions

Almost any position can be used: face-to-face, with your lover's legs pulled forward; you behind her, *him* as she kneels or stands or lies face away from you; your lover on her *his* side, with you sitting up, so it's a half-rear, half-side entry position; you lying on your back, with your lover straddling your hips on top. Go with whichever position your lover feels most comfortable with. *WHATEVER GETS MY BFHC IN*

Health Considerations

You should take into account that sperm can leak from her anus and impregnate her. Remember that the anus and vagina are very close together.

Lastly, always wear a condom. AIDS aside, the anus is not padded with the thick lining the vagina has. Small tears occur in the lining of the anus. In addition, very virulent bacteria live in the anus. Once you engage in anal intercourse, you must wash your penis before inserting it in her vagina. The bacteria in the anus can cause a terrible infection if it comes in contact with the vagina.

21 | *Kinky Sex*

Kinky sex is a term that covers a wide range of activities—from the relatively benign, such as shaving off your public hair, to the downright dangerous behavior that can take place during sadomasochism.

Kinky sex becomes deviant behavior when it is a habitual part of your sexual experiences. If unusual sex is necessary for you to be sexually satisfied, you must make sure you find lovers who feel similarly. If it's your lover who seems attached to certain behavior, then you must decide if you want to continue in a relationship that will include such acts.

Don't be frightened away from kinky sex for fear that you'll be addicted once you try it. You have to work at it to make it a habit. Just keep in mind that kinky sex is only exciting if it's unusual. If you get hung up on one kink, then you have defeated the object of kinky sex.

Even on an occasional basis, kinky sex is a highly personal thing. One person's thrill will disgust someone else. You must be sure that you have a meeting of minds with your lover. Never pressure your lover to do something she doesn't want to do, never allow yourself to do something that bothers you. If you have reservations, then don't do it. But don't let your fear of what your lover will think or what is "right" keep you from suggesting it. You may be surprised at her reaction. After all, if you try something, and it leaves you both cold, then you won't ever have to do it again.

Just remember—you and your lover are free to explore any

area you find intriguing or interesting. If you just want to add some spice to your sex life or are curious about the possibilities (and your partner is agreeable) then go ahead. Have fun!

Pubic Hair

To shave or not to shave. Many men are turned on by the sight of bare genitals—both their own and their lover's.

The act of removing the public hair can be erotic. To shave off pubic hair, cut the hair close before shaving. Use soap as a lubricant and be very careful.

Shaving can have an unfortunate side effect, however. Many people find that it is unbearably painful or irritating when the stubble grows in. If this is the case, you have no choice but to grow the hair out again. It's too sensitive an area to allow irritation to continue.

Pain

Some people find that pain can enhance sexual pleasure. Whether it's fingernails dragged across the skin or love bites, if it is pleasurable to both partners then there is no problem.

However, if it is important for you to seriously inflict or receive pain while having sex, you need to find a partner who enjoys your preference.

Spanking

In spanking, the pain inflicted is not as important as the sense of shame in the one spanked and the domination of the one doing the spanking. *Hmm SPANKING*

Habitual spankers usually have a ritual of "misbehavior" that gives them an excuse for exercising "punishment." In effect, spanking is a controlled sort of violence.

Yes some spanking For the naughty MR DANcy

Bondage

Essential to bondage is the knowledge that one of you is in complete control and the other must submit. It's foolish to engage in bondage with a stranger or someone you don't trust.

Bondage can be exciting if it is spontaneous and an unusual event. Premeditated bondage falls into the deviant category rather than kinky sex, and will affect your relationship outside of sex.

Cross-Dressing

If you have a secret yen to put on women's high heels and underwear, why not try it? Don't be worried about what your lover may think. Many women are intrigued by the feminine side of men, and have tried to put makeup on their boyfriends or held a dress up to their lover to see the effect.

Rubber

Rubber has peculiar sensual qualities. It's stretchy, it has a distinctive smell, and it clings. You'll never know until you try if it turns you on.

Do you have a rubber raincoat? That's the cheapest way to experiment with rubber. Some people are even turned on by the rubbery texture of condoms.

Urination

Some people get a thrill from watching their lover or being watched by their lover as they pass water. Many women are simply curious about how men urinate, just as they are curious in general about the workings of a man's penis.

When it comes to urinating on your lover, that's something you both will have to agree to. Yes

Ménage à trois   *No*

The appeal and success of a threesome depends on the people involved. If it's not what you want, or not what your lover wants, then it won't work.

Can you stand the thought of sharing your lover with another man? If you can't, even if you convince her to share you with another woman, you'll be doing your relationship irreparable harm. But if there's no jealousy in sight and all parties are willing, then ménage à trois can be very exciting.

Which is better—a man and two women, or two men and a woman? Of course, it depends on the people involved. And even though there are two people of the same sex involved, that doesn't necessarily mean they will actually engage in sex. There is often more voyeurism and exhibitionism involved in ménage à trois than anything homoerotic.

Orgies

An orgy is a larger version of the ménage à trois and even harder to bring off—especially if your lover is involved. If you just want to pair off with one person during an orgy, you haven't got the concept and shouldn't be involved.

You must be willing to have sex with people you might not really know, in front of other people you might not really know. Unless you happen to be sexually ready and willing to go when an orgy begins, it's usually a question of keeping an open mind until you are carried away by the whole thing.

If you can leave your inhibitions behind you, it can be an erotic, memorable experience.

22 | *Sexual Aids*

Sexual aids are objects that are used to enhance your sexual encounters, whether it's sexy clothing, satin sheets, erotica, toys, or aphrodisiacs. Almost anything can be used to add variety to sex—and since monotony is often the death of sex, don't you think you should explore some of these options?

Clothing

Sexy clothing is an excellent way to vary your sexual experience. Buy your lover pretty, sexy bits of lingerie. Don't be embarrassed about going into a store to do this—most saleswomen love it when a man comes in to buy his lover such a thoughtful gift. They wish their lover would do the same thing.

And don't be worried about your lover's reaction, either. Give her your gift, and tell her, "You're so beautiful and sexy, I wanted to buy something beautiful for you." Even if it doesn't fit or is the wrong color, your lover will be deeply touched.

As your relationship progresses, the two of you can choose sexy clothing together. This can be an erotic experience in itself. Mail order catalogs are especially good for this since you can follow through on the titillation right then and there. Remember when you go through the catalog together to always bring the focus back on your lover. This isn't a *Penthouse* magazine, where you can point and say,

"Wow, look at her!" Instead, tell your lover how good the clothing would look on her, and that you just can't wait to see her in it.

And don't forget yourself. You don't have to run out and buy a leather codpiece to be sexy—unless you want to! But pay attention to what your lover says about you. Does she like your arms? Then wear sleeveless T-shirts. Does she like your chest? Then take off your shirt when you are together around the house. Your legs? Wear shorts or just a T-shirt. Use clothing to accent the qualities your lover enjoys about your body and you won't ever go wrong.

Substances

Lotion or oil applied to the skin can be very erotic. It eases the friction from skin contact, and makes your touch much more sensual.

You can also use edible substance, like whipping cream, chocolate syrup, honey, etc. Pour some on—anywhere—and lick it off. Then let her have a treat. Sensational!

Aphrodisiacs

Erotic power has been ascribed to hundreds of drinks and foods at one time or another—oysters, quail eggs, ginger, chocolate, and more. However, most of these items are useful because of their association with sex, rather than the physical effect of arousing sexuality.

Even Spanish fly, or cantharides, the most famous aphrodisiac, doesn't create a sexual reaction in your body. In fact, many of the powders and mixtures sold as aphrodisiacs aren't healthy and can be very dangerous. Don't even try these things.

Alcohol can remove your inhibitions, but too much can have the reverse effect of an aphrodisiac. Your sensations become blunted and your erection can become chancy.

Marijuana is a mood enhancer, so if you are feeling sexy, it can make intercourse very interesting. For some people, marijuana is far too relaxing to make for good sex.

Ecstasy is reputed to enhance the sexual experience. However, its long-term effects are unknown.

Cocaine, like every other drug, can have different effects on people, depending on their body chemistry. Some men swear by cocaine, saying it prolongs and enhances the sexual experience. But it's also true that cocaine tends to wreack havoc with your erection.

Sex Toys

As with any other gimmick, you can rapidly tire of using sex toys. But even if they give you a couple of nights of amusement and sexy fun, they're worth it.

Vibrators

Vibrators and dildos are probably the most common sex toys. Vibrators are great, for both men and women. You hold it against your genitals—or rub it anywhere on your body to feel its tingling, relaxing vibration.

A vibrator can be used alone or with your partner. You'll be doing yourself and your lover a big service by buying her a vibrator. It's an excellent way for women to learn how to climax. Contrary to popular belief, a woman can't become addicted to her vibrator—the more she learns her own responses and it feels to climax, the easier it will be for her to climax at other times.

Dildos

strap on

Dildos are stiff, phallic-shaped objects that are used for vaginal or anal stimulation. The size depends on which area it is to be used for.

If you use a homemade dildo, make certain it is clean, whether it's a cucumber or a bottle of ketchup. Always have a cap on empty bottles. The in-and-out movement can cause strong suction to develop, and you may find that you can't remove the bottle without causing damage to the woman's uterus.

Ben-wa Balls

Ben-wa balls, or Japanese love balls, are another sex toy. They are two weighted balls attached together that a woman inserts into her vagina. They are supposed to vibrate as the woman moves. Most women find the effect to be less than they hoped for.

Cock Rings

A cock ring is a circle of flexible material that is placed at the base of the penis. As your penis becomes erect, the cock ring traps the blood, keeping it hard for much longer. However, some men find it painful.

Erotica

Erotica is sexually oriented books, pictures, and movies. Many people enjoy using any or all of these forms of erotica as an occasional stimulant prior to or during sex.

Movies

With the advent of the VCR, it is very common and convenient to rent X-rated movies and view them at home. X-rated movies can be taken in a humorous light, yet the sight of other people engaging in sex—no matter how artificially—can be stimulating. But, as with anything, constant repetition will ruin the experience.

Magazines

Erotic magazines feature still pictures of nude men or women. Some show various forms of intercourse. Like videos, these can be both humorous and stimulating. They are especially useful for masturbation.

Some women feel insecure if they find out that you look at

these sorts of magazines. If that happens, then the best thing to do is include your lover. Flip through the magazine with her and point out the pictures you like. Tell her why—you've always wanted to sex in this position or you're attracted to large breasts. But always bring it back to your lover. Tell her that this woman reminds you of her, or this woman isn't as pretty as she is. Your lover won't ever feel as intimidated by your sex magazines again.

Books

Erotic books range from material written hundreds of years ago to the flimsy bodice rippers of today. Books are a more singular activity than pictures, but reading such literature can only expand your knowledge and acceptance of sex. Buy erotic books for your lover. Anaïs Nin is an excellent choice. Her books don't include dirty words, and are written from a woman's point of view, which your lover will appreciate.

Using Your VCR Camera

Home movies were never like this! Buy or rent a video camera and let the fun begin.

Don't just leap into filming your lover in bed. First you have to get her used to the feeling of being under the camera's eye. Once she's comfortable, then you can film her getting out of the shower, putting on her lotion, dressing to go out. The options are endless. She'll love being the center of attention.

You can also film yourselves during sex. It can add a real spark, knowing that your every move is being captured. You'll be surprised at the result. You don't have to be a great actor—your real reactions and feelings will come through better than any performance you might put on.

Filming yourselves is just half of the fun. Watch the film with your lover as foreplay for your next sexual encounter. It's better than a porno flick anytime!

23 | *Sex or Making Love?*

Sex ~~or making love?~~ When you drive your woman wild in bed, which is it?

This book has covered everything from various positions for intercourse to contraception, from kinky sex to romance. Oral sex, anal sex, massage, petting, orgasm, physique, and more. Is this sex or is it making love?

If you've read carefully, you've noticed that the only way to be great lover is by paying attention to what your lover wants and needs from you. If you care about your lover enough to try to please her, then she'll always see it as "making love," even when it's at its wildest and raunchiest.

You'll find it impossible to simply imitate the suggestions in this book if you don't feel a genuine affection for your lover. No matter how good sex is for you, you won't be driving your woman wild in bed until you really care about her. The amount of affection you have for each other will ultimately determine her satisfaction.

So, if you've got the love, I hope this book has helped give you the encouragement you need to go beyond your old habits and begin exploring the endless possibilities of a satisfying, exciting, and loving sexual relationship.

Index

85

86

Talking, 6-7, 8-11, 62
  and criticism, 9-10
  inhibitions and, 10-11
  and jealousy, 10
  romance, 6-7
Teaching, 13-14
Testis, 20
Timing, 60-61
Tongue techniques, 43-44
Touching, 5-6, 16-17, 18-19,
  44, 45, 50-51
  See also Massage;
    Masturbation; Stroking

Urethra, 15, 16
Urination, 74
Uterus, 17

Vagina, 17-18, 51
VCR camera, 80
Vibrators, 78
Vulva, 15-16, 50-51

More Sexy Books From Carol Publishing Group

Ask for any of the books listed below at your bookstore. Or to order direct from the publisher, call 1-800-447-BOOK (MasterCard or Visa), or send a check or money order for the books purchased (plus $4.00 shipping and handling for the first book ordered and 75¢ for each additional book) to Carol Publishing Group, 120 Enterprise Avenue, Dept. 1331, Secaucus, NJ 07094.

Did She or Didn't She?: Behind the Bedroom Doors of 201 Famous Women—Mart Martin
Paper $9.95 (#51669)

Driving Your Woman Wild in Bed: A Learning Annex Book—Susan Wright, ed.   Paper $8.95 (#51331)

Erotic Games: Bringing Intimacy and Passion Back Into Sex and Relationships—Gerald Schoenewolf, Ph.D.
Cloth $16.95 (#72284)

Erotic Power: An Exploration of Dominance and Submission—Gini Graham Scott, Ph.D.   Paper $10.95 (#50968)

Erotic Tales: From the Marquis de Sade to Erica Jong and Everyone in Between—Ilona "Ciccolina" Staller, ed.
Paper $10.95 (#51474)

The 50 Most Erotic Films of All Time—Maitland McDonagh   Paper $19.95 (#51697)

The Power of Fantasy: Illusion and Eroticism in Everyday Life—Gini Graham Scott   Cloth $19.95 (#72239)

Sex Facts: A Handbook for the Carnally Curious—Leslee Welch
Paper $7.95 (#51678)

Sex in Films—Parker Tyler
Oversized paper 8 1/2 " x 11", with hundreds of explicit photos $16.95 (#51465)

Sex in the Movies—Sam Frank
Oversized paper 8 1/2 " x 11", with hundreds of explicit photos $14.95 (#51115)

Sex Talk—James Wolfe, ed.
Paper $10.95 (#51564)

Total Exposure: The Movie Buff's Guide to Celebrity Nude Scenes—Jami Bernard   Paper $17.95 (#51619)

Turning Your Man Into Putty In Your Hands: A Learning Annex Book—Susan Wright   Paper $8.95 (#51455)

Red Stripe Books: The Best in Erotic Literature (all paperbacks)

• Amorous Adventures—$4.50 • **Begging For More**—$4.50 • **Carnal Cornucopia**—$4.95 • **Diplomatic Pleasures**—$4.50 • **Diplomatic Secrets**—$4.50 • **The Domino Tattoo**—$4.50 • **Elena**—$4.50 • **Eros in Paris**—$4.50 • **Exotic Nights**—$4.50 • **Further Adventures of Sharon**—$4.95 • **Hard Riding Margot**—$4.50 • **Intimate Interviews**—$4.50 • **The Japanese Way of Love**—$3.95 • **Lady Rakehell**—$4.50 • **Laure-Ann Toujours**—$4.50 • **Marcy's Year**—$4.50 • **Memoirs of a Russian Princess**—$3.95 • **Myra's Lightning**—$4.50 • **My Sex, My Soul**—$3.95 • Rocky Road to Lesbos—$4.95 • **Secret Web**—$4.50 • **Sensual Secrets**—$4.50 • Sharon—$4.50 • **Such Sweet Thunder**—$4.50 • **A Sunday Green**—$4.50 • **The Tale of Susan Aked**—$4.50 • **The Theatre of Her Mind**—$4.50 • **The Theatre of Her Mind II**—$4.50 • **The Two Sisters**—$3.95 • **Violette**—$4.50 • **Wild Abandon**—$4.95

(Prices subject to change; books subject to availability)